Mediterranean Diet Cookbook

The Complete Guide Solution with Recipes for Weight Loss, Gain Energy and Fat Burn

CW00551464

Healthy Kitchen

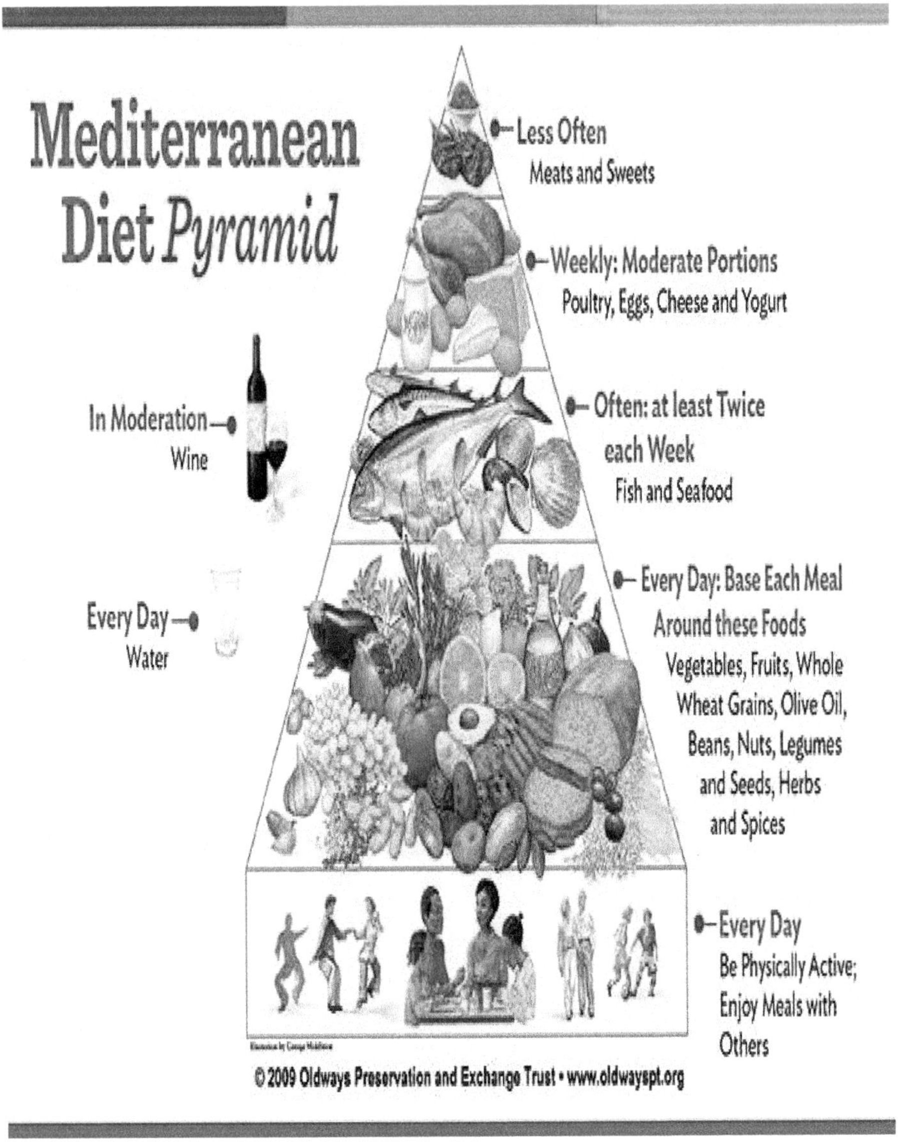
Mediterranean Diet Pyramid
Less Often
Meats and Sweets
Weekly: Moderate Portions
Poultry, Eggs, Cheese and Yogurt
In Moderation
Wine
Often: at least Twice each Week
Fish and Seafood
Every Day
Water
Every Day: Base Each Meal Around these Foods
Vegetables, Fruits, Whole Wheat Grains, Olive Oil, Beans, Nuts, Legumes and Seeds, Herbs and Spices
Every Day
Be Physically Active; Enjoy Meals with Others
© 2009 Oldways Preservation and Exchange Trust • www.oldwayspt.org

liable for any hardship or damages that may befall them after undertaking information described herein.

Additionally, the information in the following pages is intended only for informational purposes and should thus be thought of as universal. As befitting its nature, it is presented without assurance regarding its prolonged validity or interim quality. Trademarks that are mentioned are done without written consent and can in no way be considered an endorsement from the trademark holder.

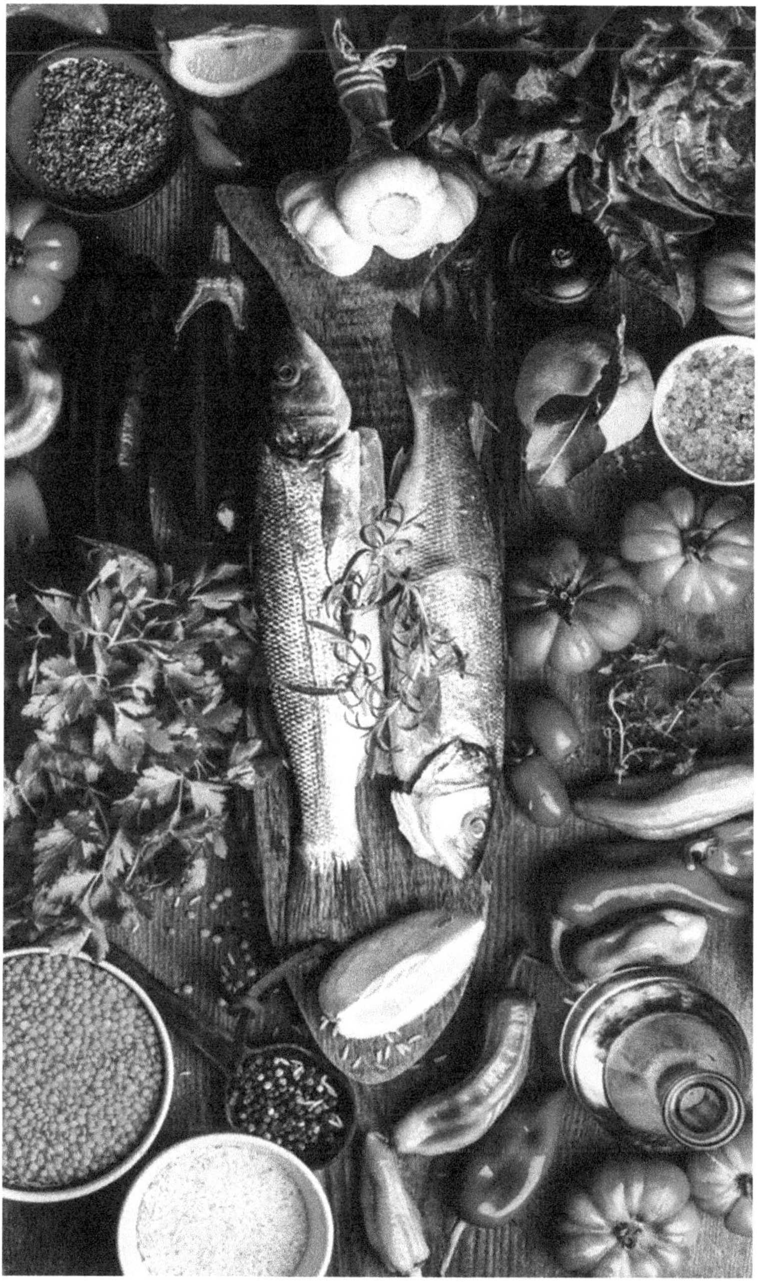

Sommario

INTRODUCTION

The Mediterranean Diet's History

While this diet was first brought to light in 1945, until the 1990s, when people started to grow a newfound knowledge of what they were eating, it did not really reach mainstream levels. This is about the time when fitness programs started to surface on TV and healthy eating started to become popular again. The Mediterranean diet is based on the premise that there is a much lower risk of heart disease among people in these regions than in people with comparable fat consumption in other areas of the world. For instance, year after year, a person living in the United States and a person living in Greece might consume the exact same amount of fat, but the American would have a greater risk of suffering from heart disease because certain elements of his or her diet are missing.

Start your Diet

Stay Hydrated

Once you've started and are fully immersed in the Mediterranean diet, you might notice that you've started to feel a little bit weak, and a little bit colder, than you're used to.

The Mediterranean diet places an emphasis on trying to cut out as much sodium from your diet as possible, which is very healthy for some of us who already have high sodium levels. Sodium, obviously is found in salt, and so we proceed to cut out salt – and then drink enough water to drain every last drop of sodium from our bodies. When it comes to hydration, the biological mechanisms for keeping us saturated and quenched rely on an equal balance of sodium and potassium. Sodium can be found in your interstitial fluid, and potassium can be found inside our cytoplasm – two sides of one wall. When you drink tons of water, sweat a lot at the gym, or both, your sodium leaves your body in your urine and your sweat. Potassium, on the other hand, is only really lost through the urine – and even then, it's rare. This means that our bodies almost constantly need a refill on our sodium levels.

Vitamins and Supplements

Vitamins and minerals can be found in plants and animals, yes, but more often than not fruits and vegetables are much stronger sources. When consume another animal, we are consuming the sum total of all of the energy and nutrition that that animal has also consumed. This might sound like a sweet deal, but the pig you're eating used that energy in his own daily life, and therefore only has a tiny bit left to offer you. Plants, on the other hand, are first-hand sources of things like calcium, vitamin K, and vitamin C, which our bodies require daily doses of.

Meal Preparation and Portion Planning

If you haven't heard of the term "meal prep" before now, it's a beautiful day to learn something that will save you time, stress, and inches on your waistline. Meal prep, short for meal preparation, is a habit that was developed mostly by the body building community in order to accurately track your macronutrients. The basic idea behind meal prep is that each weekend, you manage your free time around cooking and preparing all of your meals for the upcoming week. While most meal preppers do their grocery shopping and cooking on Sundays, to keep their meals the freshest, you can choose to cook on a Saturday if that works better with your schedule. Meal prep each week uses one large grocery list of bulk ingredients to get all the supplies you need to make four dinners and four lunches of your choice. This means that you might have to do a bit of mental math quadrupling the serving size, but all you have to do is multiply each ingredient by four. Although you don't have to meal prep more than one meal with four portions each week, if you're already in the kitchen, you most likely have cooking time to work on something else.

Tracking Your Macronutrients

Wouldn't it be nice if you could have a full nutritional label for each of your home-cooked meals, just to make sure that your numbers are adding up in favor of weight loss? Oddly enough, tracking your macronutrients in order to calculate the nutritional value of each of your meals and portions is as easy as stepping on the scale. Not the scale in your bathroom, however. A food scale! If you've never had a good relationship with your weight and numbers, you might suddenly find that they aren't too bad after all. Food scales are used to measure, well, your food, but there's a slick system of online calculators and fitness applications for your smart phone that can take this number and turn it into magic. When you meal prep each week, keep track of your recipes diligently. Remember how you multiplied each of the ingredients on the list by four to create four servings? You're going to want to remember how much of each vegetable, fruit, grain, nut, and fat you cooked with. While you wait for your meal to finish cooking, find a large enough plastic container to fit all of your meals. Make sure it's clean and dry, and use the empty container to zero out your scale.

Counting Calories and Forming a Deficit

When it comes down to the technical science, there is one way and only one way to lose weight: by eating fewer calories in one day than your body requires to survive. Now, this doesn't mean that you can't lose weight for other reasons – be it water weight, as a result of stress, or simply working out harder. Although counting calories might not be the most fun way to lose weight, a calorie deficit is the only sure-fire way of guaranteeing that you reap all the weight loss benefits of the Mediterranean diet for your efforts. Scientifically, you already know that the healthy rate of weight loss for the average adult is between one and two pounds per week.

Get ready for a little bit more math, but it's nothing you can't handle in the name of a smaller waistline. One pound of fat equals around thirty-five hundred Calories, which means that your caloric deficit needs to account for that number, each week, without making too much of a dent on your regular nutrition. For most of us, we're used to eating between fifteen hundred and two thousand calories per day, which gives you a blessedly simply five hundred calorie deficit per day in order to reach your healthy weight loss goals. If you cut out exactly five hundred calories each day, you should be able to lose one pound of fat by the end of seven days. Granted, this estimate does take into account thirty minutes of daily exercise, but the results are still about the same when you rely on the scientific facts. If your age, height, weight, and sex predispose you to eat either more or less calories per day, you might want to consult with your doctor about the healthiest way for you to integrate a caloric deficit into your Mediterranean diet.

Goal Setting to Meet Your Achievements

On the subject of control, there are a few steps and activities that you should go through before you begin your Mediterranean diet just to make sure that you have clear and realistic goals in mind. Sitting down to set goals before embarking on a totally new diet routine will help you stay focused and committed during your Mediterranean diet. While a Mediterranean diet lifestyle certainly isn't as demanding as some of the crazy diet fads you see today, it can be a struggle to focus on eating natural fruits and vegetables that are more "salt of the Earth" foods than we're used to. You already know that when it comes to weight loss, you shouldn't expect to lose more than one to two pounds per week healthily while you're dieting. You are still welcome to set a weight loss goal with time in mind, but when it comes to the Mediterranean diet, you should set your goals for one month in the future.

Losing Weight

Further studies have provided examples of weight loss from the Mediterranean diet, as 322 individuals participated in an experiment where some individuals were exposed to a low-carb diet, others undertook a low-fat diet, and some consumed only a Mediterranean diet. The findings found that those on the Mediterranean diet had the greatest weight loss of all with 12 and 10 pounds respectively being lost by the top two participants. The study stressed that weight loss from the Mediterranean diet is successful and should be considered by anyone who has difficulty losing weight.

BREAKFAST RECIPES

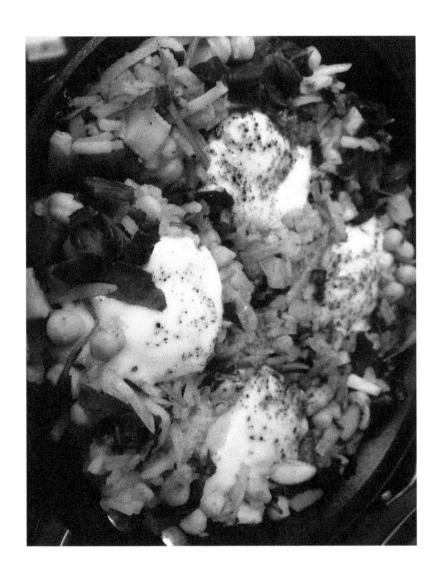

Hash of Potato and Chickpea

Ingredients:

- 4 cups of frozen hash brown potatoes shredded
- For 1 tbsp. Ginger, freshly minced,
- 1⁄2 cup of onion chopped
- 2 cups of chopped spinach for babies
- For 1 tbsp. The Curry Powder
- 1⁄2 tsp. The Salt of the Sea
- 1⁄4 cup of Virgin Olive Oil Extra
- 1 cup of zucchini chopped
- 1 (15-ounce) of canned, rinsed chickpeas
- 4 eggs of large size

Directions:

1. Combine the potatoes, ginger, onion, spinach, curry powder, and sea salt in a large cup.
2. Heat the extra virgin olive oil in a nonstick skillet set over medium-high heat and add the potato mixture.

3. Press the mixture into a layer and cook, without stirring, for around 5 minutes or until golden brown and crispy.
4. Lower to medium-low heat and fold in the zucchini and chickpeas until just blended, breaking up the mixture.

5. Briefly stir, squeeze the mixture back into a layer, and make four wells. Into each indentation, split one egg.
6. Cook for about 5 minutes, sealed, or until the eggs are set.

Mediterranean Pancakes

Ingredients:

- Old-fashioned oats for 1 cup
- 1⁄2 cup of all-use flour
- For 2 tbsp. Seeds of flax
- For 1 tsp. Soda baking
- 1⁄4 tsp. The Salt of the Sea
- For 2 tbsp. extra virgin olive oil
- 2 oversized eggs
- 2 cups of plain Greek yogurt without fat
- For 2 tbsp. Raw honey Raw honey
- Fruit, syrup, or other new toppings

Directions:

1. Combine the oats, flour, flax seeds, baking soda, and sea salt in a blender; mix for 30 seconds or so.
2. Add extra virgin olive oil, eggs, honey and yogurt and continue to pulsate until very smooth.
3. For at least 20 minutes or until dense, let the mixture stand.

4. Over medium heat, position a large nonstick skillet and brush with extra virgin olive oil.

5. Ladle the batter into the skillet in batches of quarter-cupful's.

6. Cook the pancakes for about 2 minutes or until bubbles form and golden brown.

7. Turn them over and cook for 2 more minutes or until the other sides are golden brown.

8. Put the cooked pancakes on a baking sheet and keep them warm in the oven.

9. Serve with the preferred toppings.

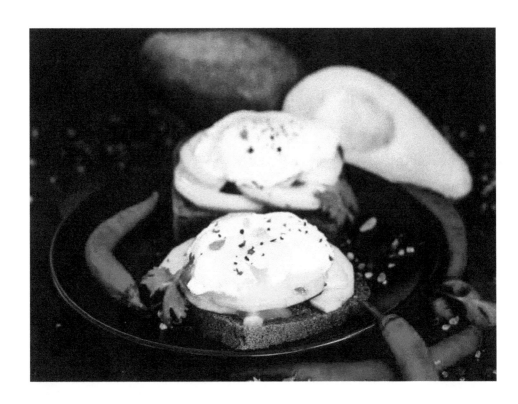

Avocado Egg Toast

Ingredients:

- 2 mature avocados, peeled
- New lemon juice squeezed, to taste
- For 2 tbsp. Mint that has been freshly chopped, plus extra to garnish
- Black pepper and sea salt, to taste
- 4 big rye bread slices
- 80 grams of Crumbled Fluffy Feta
- 1 Egg

Directions:

1. Mash the avocado roughly with a fork in a medium bowl; add lemon juice and mint and continue mashing until just mixed.
2. Season with to taste, black pepper and sea salt. Grill the bread or toast it until golden.
3. On every slice of the toasted bread, spread around 1/4 of the avocado mixture and top with feta and a cooked egg.
4. Garnish with additional mint and immediately serve.

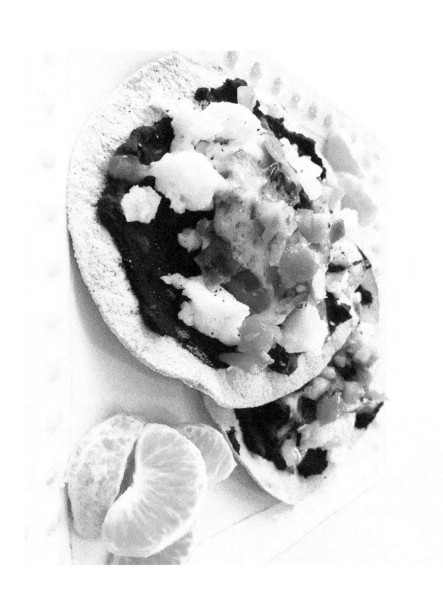

Breakfast Tostadas

Ingredients:

- ½ white onion, diced
- 1 tomato, chopped
- 1 cucumber, chopped
- 1 tablespoon fresh cilantro, chopped
- ½ jalapeno pepper, chopped
- 1 tablespoon lime juice
- 6 corn tortillas
- 1 tablespoon canola oil
- 2 oz Cheddar cheese, shredded
- ½ cup white beans, canned, drained
- 6 eggs
- ½ teaspoon butter
- ½ teaspoon Sea salt

Directions:

1. Make Pico de Galo: in the salad bowl combine together diced white onion, tomato, cucumber, fresh cilantro, and jalapeno pepper.

2. Then add lime juice and a ½ tablespoon of canola oil. Mix up the mixture well. Pico de Galo is cooked.
3. After this, preheat the oven to 390F.
4. Line the tray with baking paper.
5. Arrange the corn tortillas on the baking paper and brush with remaining canola oil from both sides.
6. Bake for 10 minutes.
7. Chill the cooked crunchy tortillas well.
8. Meanwhile, toss the butter in the skillet.
9. Crack the eggs in the melted butter and sprinkle them with sea salt.
10. Fry the eggs for 3-5 minutes over the medium
11. heat.
12. After this, mash the beans until you get puree
13. texture.
14. Spread the bean puree on the corn tortillas.
15. Add fried eggs.
16. Then top the eggs with Pico de Galo and shredded Cheddar cheese.

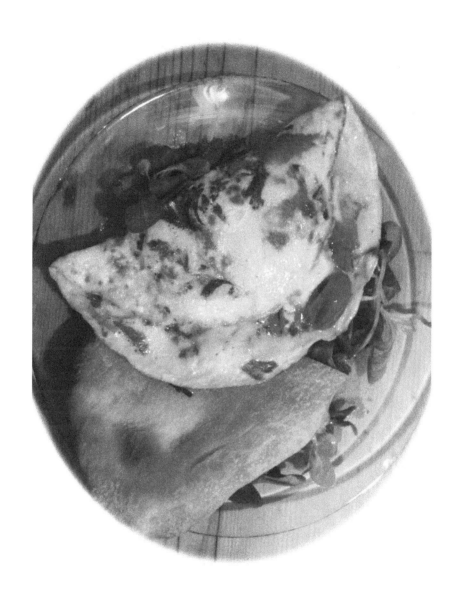

Parmesan Omelet

Ingredients:

- 1 tablespoon cream cheese
- 2 eggs, beaten
- ¼ teaspoon paprika
- ½ teaspoon dried oregano
- ¼ teaspoon dried dill
- 1 oz Parmesan, grated
- 1 teaspoon coconut oil

Directions:

1. Mix up together cream cheese with eggs, dried oregano, and dill.
2. Preheat coconut oil in the skillet.
3. Place egg mixture in the skillet and flatten it.
4. Add grated Parmesan and close the lid.
5. Cook omelet for 10 minutes over the low heat.
6. Then transfer the cooked omelet in the serving plate and sprinkle with paprika.

Menemen

Ingredients:

- 2 tomatoes, chopped
- 2 eggs, beaten
- 1 bell pepper, chopped
- 1 teaspoon tomato paste
- ¼ cup of water
- 1 teaspoon butter
- ½ white onion, diced
- ½ teaspoon chili flakes
- 1/3 teaspoon sea salt

Directions:

1.   Put butter in the pan and melt it.

2.   Add bell pepper and cook it for 3 minutes over the medium heat. Stir it from time to time.

3.   After this, add diced onion and cook it for 2 minutes more.

4.   Stir the vegetables and add tomatoes.

5.   Cook them for 5 minutes over the medium-low heat.

6.   Then add water and tomato paste. Stir well.

7.   Add beaten eggs, chili flakes, and sea salt.

8.   Stir well and cook menemen for 4 minutes over the medium-low heat.

9.   The cooked meal should be half runny.

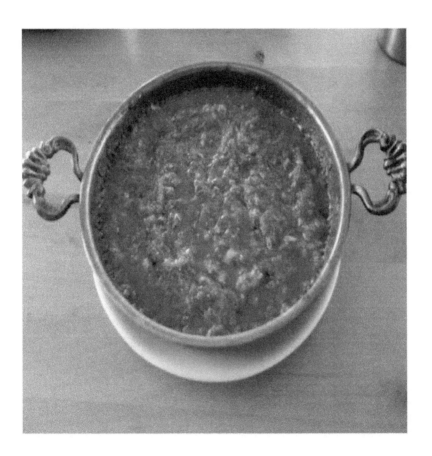

Watermelon Pizza

Ingredients:

- 9 oz watermelon slice
- 1 tablespoon Pomegranate sauce
- 2 oz Feta cheese, crumbled
- 1 tablespoon fresh cilantro, chopped

Directions:

1. Place the watermelon slice in the plate and sprinkle with crumbled Feta cheese.
2. Add fresh cilantro.
3. After this, sprinkle the pizza with Pomegranate juice generously.
4. Cut the pizza into the servings.

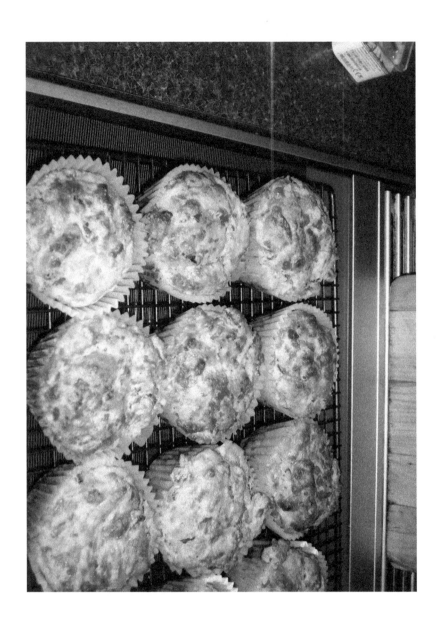

Ham Muffins

Ingredients:

- 3 oz ham, chopped
- 4 eggs, beaten
- 2 tablespoons coconut flour
- ½ teaspoon dried oregano
- ¼ teaspoon dried cilantro
- Cooking spray

Directions:

1. Spray the muffin's molds with cooking spray from inside.
2. In the bowl mix up together beaten eggs, coconut flour, dried oregano, cilantro, and ham.
3. When the liquid is homogenous, pour it in the prepared muffin molds.
4. Bake the muffins for 15 minutes at 360F.
5. Chill the cooked meal well and only after this remove from the molds.

SNACKS

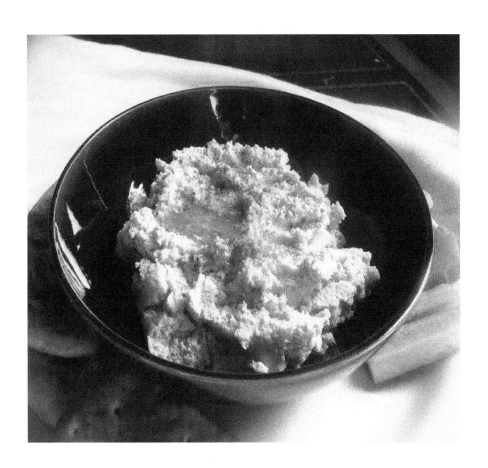

Light & Creamy Garlic Hummus

Ingredients:

- 1 1/2 cups dry chickpeas, rinsed
- 2 1/2 tbsp fresh lemon juice
- 1 tbsp garlic, minced
- 1/2 cup tahini
- 6 cups of water
- Pepper
- Salt

Directions:

1.   Add water and chickpeas into the instant pot.

2.   Seal pot with a lid and select manual and set timer for 40 minutes.

3.   Once done, allow to release pressure naturally. Remove lid.

4.   Drain chickpeas well and reserved 1/2 cup chickpeas liquid.

5.   Transfer chickpeas, reserved liquid, lemon juice, garlic, tahini, pepper, and salt into the food processor and process until smooth.

6.   Serve and enjoy.

Perfect Queso

Ingredients:

- 1 lb ground beef
- 32 oz Velveeta cheese, cut into cubes
- 10 oz can tomatoes, diced
- 1 1/2 tbsp taco seasoning
- 1 tsp chili powder
- 1 onion, diced
- Pepper
- Salt

Directions:

1. Set instant pot on sauté mode.
2. Add meat, onion, taco seasoning, chili powder, pepper, and salt into the pot and cook until meat is no longer pink.
3. Add tomatoes and stir well. Top with cheese and do not stir.
4. Seal pot with lid and cook on high for 4 minutes.
5. Once done, release pressure using quick release. Remove lid.
6. Stir everything well and serve.

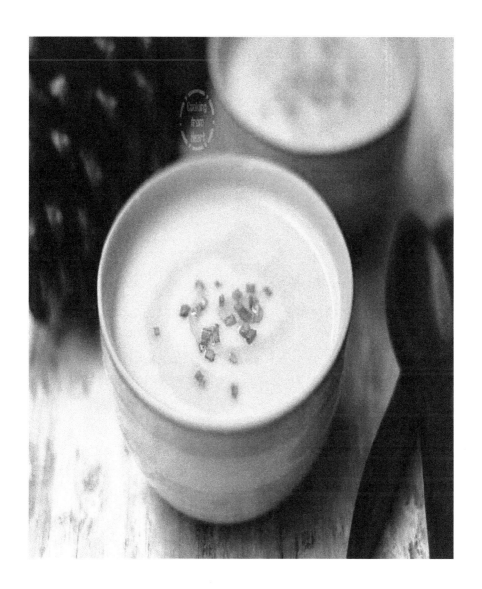

Creamy Potato Spread

Ingredients:

- 1 lb sweet potatoes, peeled and chopped 3/4 tbsp fresh chives, chopped
- 1/2 tsp paprika
- 1 tbsp garlic, minced
- 1 cup tomato puree
- Pepper
- Salt

Directions:

1. Add all ingredients except chives into the inner pot of instant pot and stir well.
2. Seal pot with lid and cook on high for 15 minutes.
3. Once done, allow to release pressure naturally for 10 minutes, then release remaining using quick release. Remove lid.
4. Transfer instant pot sweet potato mixture into the food processor and process until smooth.
5. Garnish with chives and serve.

Cucumber Tomato Okra Salsa

Ingredients:

- 1 lb tomatoes, chopped
- 1/4 tsp red pepper flakes
- 1/4 cup fresh lemon juice
- 1 cucumber, chopped
- 1 tbsp fresh oregano, chopped
- 1 tbsp fresh basil, chopped
- 1 tbsp olive oil
- 1 onion, chopped
- 1 tbsp garlic, chopped
- 1 1/2 cups okra, chopped
- Pepper
- Salt

Directions

1.   Add oil into the inner pot of instant pot and set the pot on sauté mode.

2.   Add onion, garlic, pepper, and salt and sauté for 3 minutes.

3.   Add remaining ingredients except for cucumber and stir well.

4.   Seal pot with lid and cook on high for 12 minutes.

5.   Once done, allow to release pressure naturally for 10 minutes then release remaining using quick release. Remove lid.

6.   Once the salsa mixture is cool then add cucumber and mix well.

7.   Serve and enjoy.

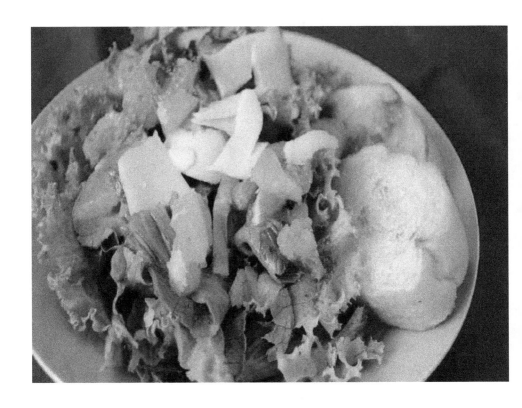

Roasted Beet Salad with Ricotta Cheese

Ingredients:

- Red beets (8.8 oz, large, wrapped in foil)
- Yellow beets (8.8 oz, small, wrapped in foil)
- Mesclun (4.3 oz)
- Mustard Vinaigrette (4.4 oz)
- Ricotta cheese (2.1 oz)
- Walnuts (0.1 oz, chopped)

Directions:

1.   Bake at 400 F for 1 hour.

2.   Cool the beets slightly. Trim the root and stem ends and pull off the peels.

3.   Cut the red beets crosswise into thin slices.

4.   Cut the yellow beets vertically into quarters.

5.   Arrange the sliced red beets in circles on cold salad plates. Toss the mesclun with half the vinaigrette.

6.   Drizzle the remaining vinaigrette over the sliced beets.

7.   Situate small mound of greens in the center of each plate.

8.   Arrange the quartered yellow beets around the greens.

9.   Sprinkle the tops of the salads with the crumbled ricotta and walnuts (if using).

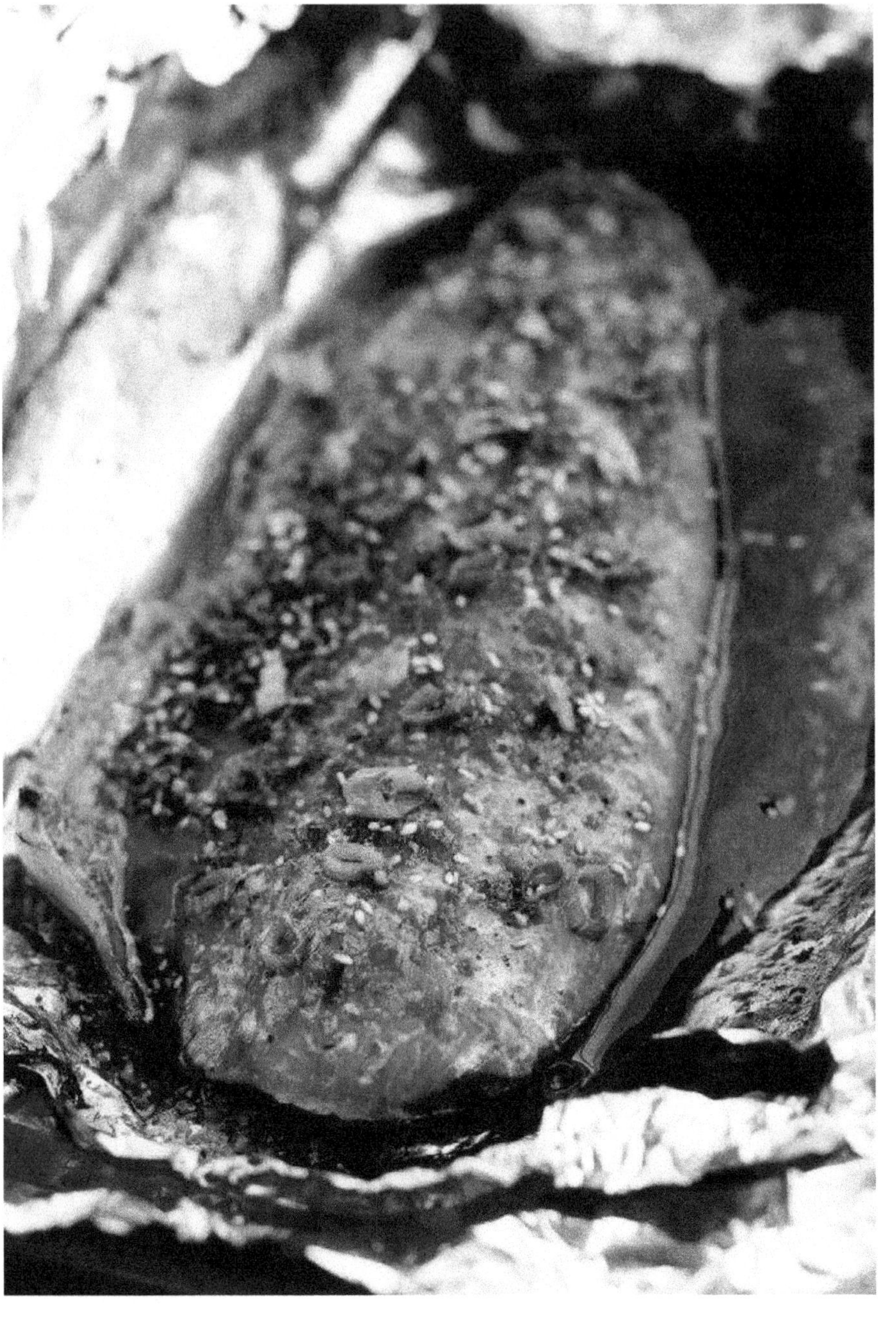

Baked Fish with Tomatoes and Mushrooms

Ingredients:

- Fish (4, whole and small, 12 oz each)
- Salt (to taste)
- Pepper (to taste)
- Dried thyme (pinch)
- Parsley (4 sprigs)
- Olive oil (as needed)
- Onion (4 oz, small dice)
- Shallots (1 oz, minced)
- Mushrooms (8 oz, chopped)
- Tomato concassed (6.4 oz)
- Dry white wine (3.2 Fl oz)

Directions:

1. Scale and clean the fish but leaves the heads on. Season the fish inside and out with salt and pepper and put a small pinch of thyme and a sprig of parsley in the cavity of each.
2. Use as many baking pans to hold the fish in a single layer. Oil the pans with a little olive oil.
3. Sauté the onions and shallots in a little olive oil about 1 minute. Add the mushrooms and sauté lightly.

4. Put the sautéed vegetables and the tomatoes in the bottoms of the baking pans.
5. Put the fish in the pans. Oil the tops lightly. Pour in the wine.
6. Bake at 400F for 15-20 minutes.
7. Remove the fish and keep them warm.
8. Remove the vegetables from the pans with a slotted spoon and check for seasonings. Serve a spoonful of the vegetables with the fish, placing it under or alongside each fish.
9. Strain, degrease, and reduce the cooking liquid slightly. Just before serving, moisten each portion with 1-2 tbsp of the juice.

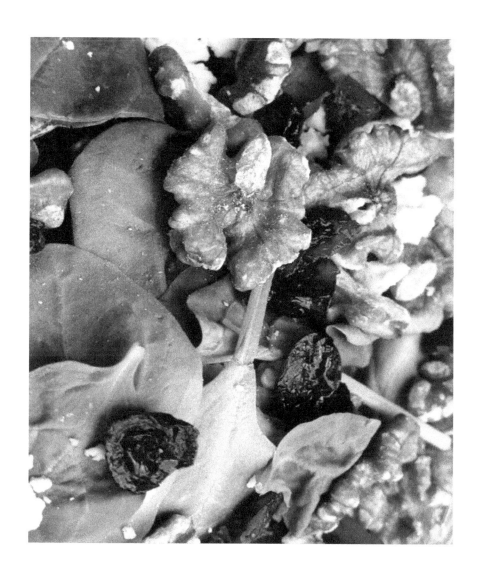

Goat Cheese and Walnut Salad

Ingredients:

- Beet (2 oz)
- Arugula (3 oz)
- Bibb lettuce (2 oz)
- Romaine lettuce (9 oz)
- Breadcrumbs (1/4 cup, dry)
- Dried thyme (1/4 tbs)
- Dried basil (1/4 tbs)
- Black pepper (1/3 tsp)
- Fresh goat's milk cheese (6.35 oz, preferably in log shape)
- Walnut pieces (1.1 oz)
- Red wine vinaigrette (2 fl. Oz.)

Directions:

1. Trim, wash, and dry all the salad greens.
2. Tear the greens into small pieces. Toss well.
3. Mix the herbs, pepper, and crumbs.
4. Slice the cheese into 1 oz pieces. In the seasoned crumbs mix, roll the pieces of cheese to coat them

5. Place the cheese on a sheet pan. Bake at the temperate of 425 F for 10 minutes.
6. Simultaneously, toast the walnuts in a dry sauté pan or the oven with the cheese.
7. Toss the greens with the vinaigrette and arrange on cold plates. Top each plate of greens with 2 pieces of cheese and sprinkle with walnuts.

Grilled Spiced Turkey Burger

Ingredients:

- Onion (1.8 oz, chopped fine)
- Extra Virgin Olive Oil (1/3 tbsp)
- Turkey (14.4 oz, ground)
- Salt (1/3 tbsp)
- Curry powder (1/3 tbsp)
- Lemon zest (2/5 tsp, grated)
- Pepper (1/8 tsp)
- Cinnamon (1/8 tsp)
- Coriander (1/4 tsp, ground)
- Cumin (1/8 tsp, ground)
- Cardamom (1/8 tsp, ground)
- Water (1.2 Fl oz)
- Tomato Raisin Chutney (as desired)
- Cilantro leaves (as desired)

Directions:

1. Cook the onions in the oil. Cool completely.
2. Combine the turkey, onions, spices, water, and salt in a bowl. Toss.

3.   Divide the mixture into 5 oz portions (or as desired). Form each part into a thick patty.

4.   Broil but do not overcook it.

5.   Plate the burgers. Put spoonful of chutney on top of each.

SALADS

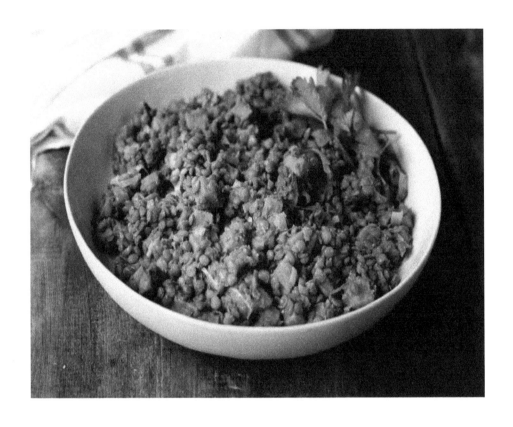

Lentil Salmon Salad

Ingredients:

- Vegetable stock - 2 cups
- Green lentils - 1, rinsed
- Red onion - 1, chopped
- Parsley - 1 2 cup, chopped
- Smoked salmon - 4 oz., shredded
- Cilantro - 2 tbsp., chopped
- Red pepper - 1, chopped
- Lemon - 1, juiced
- Salt and pepper - to taste

Directions:

1. Cook vegetable stock and lentils in a saucepan for 15 to 20 minutes, on low heat. Ensure all liquid has been absorbed and then remove from heat.
2. Pour into a salad bowl and top with red pepper, parsley, cilantro and salt and pepper (to suit your taste) and mix.
3. Mix in lemon juice and shredded salmon.
4. This salad should be served fresh.

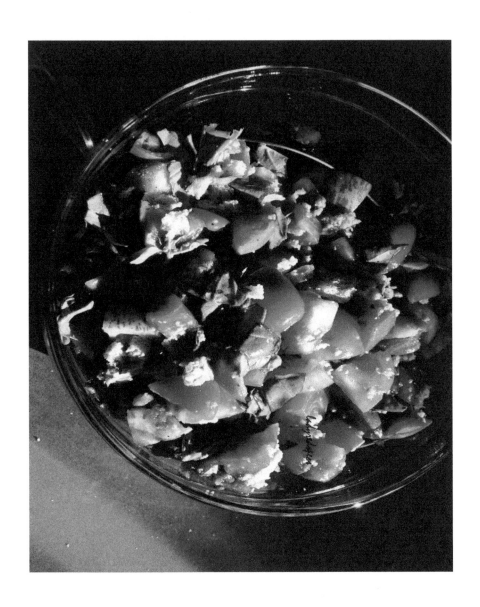

Peppy Pepper Tomato Salad

Ingredients:

- Yellow bell pepper - 1, cored and diced Cucumbers - 4, diced
- Red onion - 1, chopped
- Balsamic vinegar – 1 tbsp.
- Extra virgin olive oil – 2 tbsp.
- Tomatoes - 4, diced
- Red bell peppers - 2, cored and diced
- Chili flakes - 1 pinch
- Salt and pepper - to taste

Directions:

1. Mix all the above ingredients in a salad bowl, except salt and pepper.
2. Season with salt and pepper to suit your taste and mix well.
3. Eat while fresh.

Cashews and Red Cabbage Salad

Ingredients:

- 1-pound red cabbage, shredded
- 2 tablespoons coriander, chopped
- ½ cup cashews halved
- 2 tablespoons olive oil
- 1 tomato, cubed
- A pinch of salt and black pepper
- 1 tablespoon white vinegar

Directions:

1. Mix the cabbage with the coriander and the rest of the ingredients in a salad bowl, toss and serve cold.

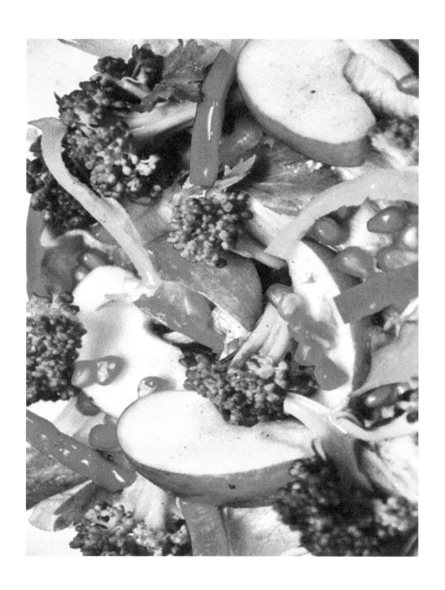

Apples and Pomegranate Salad

Ingredients:

- 3 big apples, cored and cubed
- 1 cup pomegranate seeds
- 3 cups baby arugula
- 1 cup walnuts, chopped
- 1 tablespoon olive oil
- 1 teaspoon white sesame seeds
- 2 tablespoons apple cider vinegar

Directions:

1. Mix the apples with the arugula and the rest of the ingredients in a bowl, toss and serve cold.

Cranberry Bulgur Mix

Ingredients:

- 1 and ½ cups hot water
- 1 cup bulgur
- Juice of ½ lemon
- 4 tablespoons cilantro, chopped
- ½ cup cranberries
- 1 and ½ teaspoons curry powder
- ¼ cup green onions
- ½ cup red bell peppers
- ½ cup carrots, grated
- 1 tablespoon olive oil

Directions:

1. Put bulgur into a bowl, add the water, stir, cover, leave aside for 10 minutes, fluff with a fork, and transfer to a bowl. Add the rest of the ingredients, toss, and serve cold.

Mediterranean Chopped Salad

Ingredients:

- For 2 tbsp. Olive Oil Extra Virgin Oil
- ¼ cup Kalamata olives coarsely chopped
- ¼ cup of scallions chopped
- 1 cup of diced seedless cucumber, 2 medium tomatoes,
- 1 cup of diced seedless cucumber
- ¼ cup of fresh parsley chopped
- For 1 tbsp. Vinegar from white-wine
- Pepper freshly ground
- ¼ tsp. The Salt of the Sea

Directions:

1. Get your grill preheated.
2. Combine extra virgin olive oil, lemon juice, oregano, garlic, sea salt and black pepper in a small bowl; reserve for basting two tablespoons of the mixture.
3. Rinse and drain the tofu; pat dry with paper towels. Break the crosswise tofu into 8
4. Place the 1/2-inch thick slices in a glass bowl.
5. Apply the marinade of lemon juice and turn on the tofu to coat correctly.
6. Marinate for a minimum of 30 minutes in the fridge.
7. Prepare the salad in the meantime.

8. Combine all the salad ingredients in a medium bowl; toss gently to blend well.

9. Only set aside.

10. Brush with oil on the grill rack. Drain the tofu that has been marinated and discard the marinade.

11. Grill tofu over medium heat, for around 4 minutes per hand, basting periodically with the remaining lemon juice marinade. Serve warm tofu on the grill, topped with salad.

Mediterranean Salad Barley

Ingredients:

- Two and a half cups of water, 1 cup of barley
- Oh. 4 tbsp. Virgin Olive Oil Extra, Split
- Garlic 2 cloves
- 7 tomatoes sun-dried
- For 1 tbsp. Vinegar Balsamic Vinegar
- ½ cup of black olives chopped
- ½ cup of cilantro finely chopped

Directions:

1. In a casserole, combine water and barley; bring the mixture to a rolling boil over high heat.
2. Lower heat to medium-low and simmer, covered, until soft, but still slightly firm in the centre, about 30 minutes.
3. Drain and move to a large bowl; cool to room temperature with the cooked barley.
4. Purée 2 tablespoons of extra virgin olive oil, garlic, sun-dried tomatoes and balsamic vinegar in a blender until

very smooth, then pour the remaining olive oil, olives and cilantro over the barley.

5. Refrigerate until chilled, sealed. Until eating, swirl to blend appropriately.

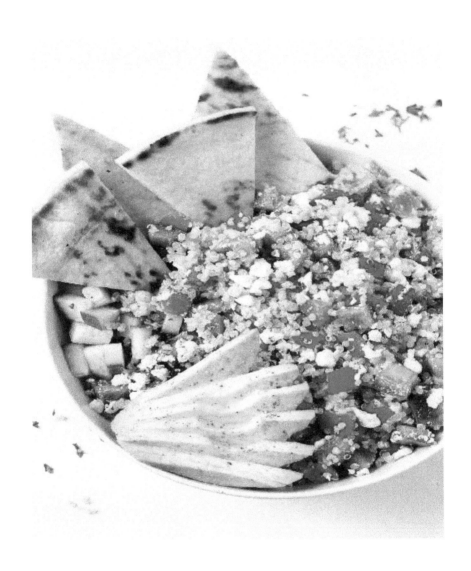

Mediterranean Quinoa Salad

Ingredients:

- 1 clove Garlic, crushed
- Water for 2 cups
- 2 chicken bouillon cubes
- 1 cup of quinoa uncooked
- 1/2 cup of chopped olives from Kalamata 1 big red onion, diced
- 2 (cooked) large chicken breasts, diced
- 1 broad bell pepper, pink, diced
- 1/2 cup of feta cheese crumbled
- 1/4 cup of fresh chives chopped
- 1/4 cup of fresh parsley chopped
- 1/2 tsp. The Salt of the Sea
- 1/4 cup of Virgin Olive Oil Extra
- For 1 tbsp. Vinegar Balsamic Vinegar
- 2/3 of a cup of fresh lemon juice

Directions:

1. In a saucepan, combine the garlic, water, and bouillon cubes; bring the mixture to a boil over medium-low heat.

---

2. Stir in the quinoa and simmer, covered, for around 20 minutes or until the quinoa is tender and the water has been absorbed.
3. Put the cooked quinoa in a large bowl and remove the garlic cloves. Combine the olives, onion, ham, bell pepper, feta cheese, chives, parsley, sea salt, extra virgin olive oil, lemon juice, and balsamic vinegar. Serve chilled or hot.

Healthy Greece Salad

Ingredients:

- 1 small red, chopped onion
- 2 cucumbers, sliced and peeled
- 3 big ripe, chopped tomatoes
- Oh. 4 tsp. Lemon Juice Freshly Squeezed
- 1/4 cup of Virgin Olive Oil Extra
- Tsp. 1 1/2. Oregano dried
- Salt from the Sea
- Black pepper Ground
- 6 black Greek olives pitted and sliced
- 1 cup of feta cheese crumbled

Directions:

1. In a shallow salad bowl, mix the onion, cucumber, and tomatoes; sprinkle with the lemon juice, extra virgin olive oil, oregano, sea salt and black pepper.
2. Sprinkle over the salad with the olives and feta and serve immediately.

MAIN DISHES

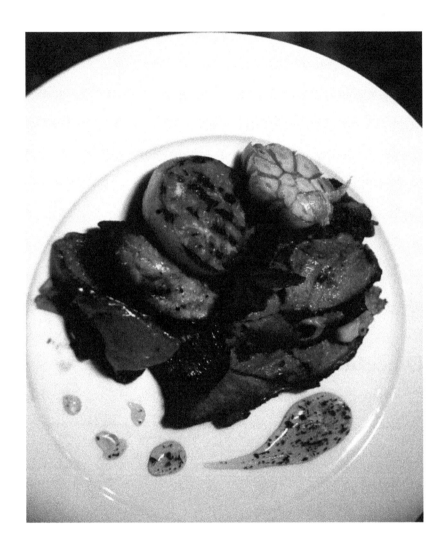

Grilled Vegetable Lamb

Ingredients:

- ⅓ cup of olive oil extra virgin
- 1 clove of fresh, minced garlic
- 1 tablespoon of mint chopped
- Salt and to taste, freshly ground pepper
- Lamb sirloin, 1½ pounds, cut into 1½-inch cubes
- 8 large leaves of bay
- 8 fresh caps with mushrooms
- 8 small tomatoes from cherry
- 1 big green bell pepper, seeded and cut into strips of 1½-inch
- 2 small zucchinis, cut into 1-inch cubes
- 4 medium onions, cut into quarters

Directions:

1. In a resealable plastic baggie, combine the lemon juice, olive oil, garlic, mint, and salt and pepper to taste and pour over the lamb cubes. Marinate overnight or for at least 8 hours and place in the refrigerator. Meat, bay leaves, and vegetables alternate on 8 flat-bladed oiled

skewers. Grill over hot coals for about 15 minutes, sometimes turning skewers.

2. A chopped salad of onions, cucumbers, tomatoes and parsley goes well with this dish. For the dressing, use lemon juice.

Stuffed Baked Trout

Ingredients:

- Extra-virgin olive oil 3 tablespoons
- 1 big, finely chopped onion
- Four cloves of fresh, minced garlic
- 2/3 cup of simple crumbs for bread
- 1 Lemon, juiced and grated with rind
- 1/3 cup dark raisins without seeds, chopped
- 1/2 cup of pine nuts
- 2 teaspoons of new chopped parsley
- 1 tablespoon fresh dill chopped
- Salt and to taste, freshly ground pepper
- 1/4 cup substitute for eggs
- 4 (12-ounce) of whole, scaled and gutted trout
- Cooking Spray with Olive Oil
- Wedges of lemon for garnish

Directions:

1. Heat 2 tablespoons of olive oil in a skillet, add the onion and garlic and cook until tender, then remove from the heat. Mix the bread crumbs, grated lemon rind, raisins,

pine nuts, parsley, dill, and salt and pepper in a wide bowl.

2. Add the garlic and egg mixture and mix well. Stuff each trout with the mixture and put it in a single layer on a shallow baking pan sprayed with oil. Make multiple diagonal slashes around each fish's body and drizzle with the remaining tablespoon of oil and lemon juice.

3. Bake for about 30-45 minutes or until the fish flakes at 375 degrees. Serve hot with a garnish of lemon wedges.

Great Northern Beans and Chicken

Ingredients:

- Skinless, boneless chicken legs 2 (3-ounce)
- Skinless, boneless chicken breasts 2 (4-ounce)
- 2 onions, sliced into big chunks
- Five carrots, one sliced and another sliced into big bits
- 2 celery stalks, 1 sliced and another one cut into large pieces.
- Cooking Spray with Olive Oil
- 2 cups of low sodium canned, fat-free chicken broth
- 4 cups of canned, drained and rinsed Great Northern beans Two tomatoes, peeled and cut into big bits,
- ½ green bell pepper, cut into large chunks 2 new teaspoons of thyme
- 3 cloves of fresh, chopped garlic
- 2 teaspoons of new chopped parsley Salt and to taste, freshly ground pepper

Directions:

1. Rinse the chicken and pat dry underwater. In a saucepan, place the chicken, half of the onions, 1 sliced carrot and 1 sliced celery stalk. To cover the chicken, add water, and cook over medium heat until the chicken is soft. Strain

yourself and set aside. Use for cooking spray to gently spray the bottom and sides of a large casserole dish and add chicken, 2 cups of broth and beans.

2. Along with the tomatoes, add the remaining carrot and celery parts to the casserole, the remaining onion, green bell pepper, thyme, garlic, parsley, salt and pepper. Bake for 45 minutes, until mixture simmers. While hot, serve.

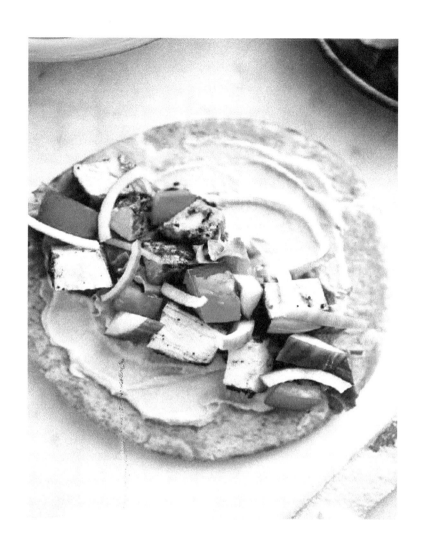

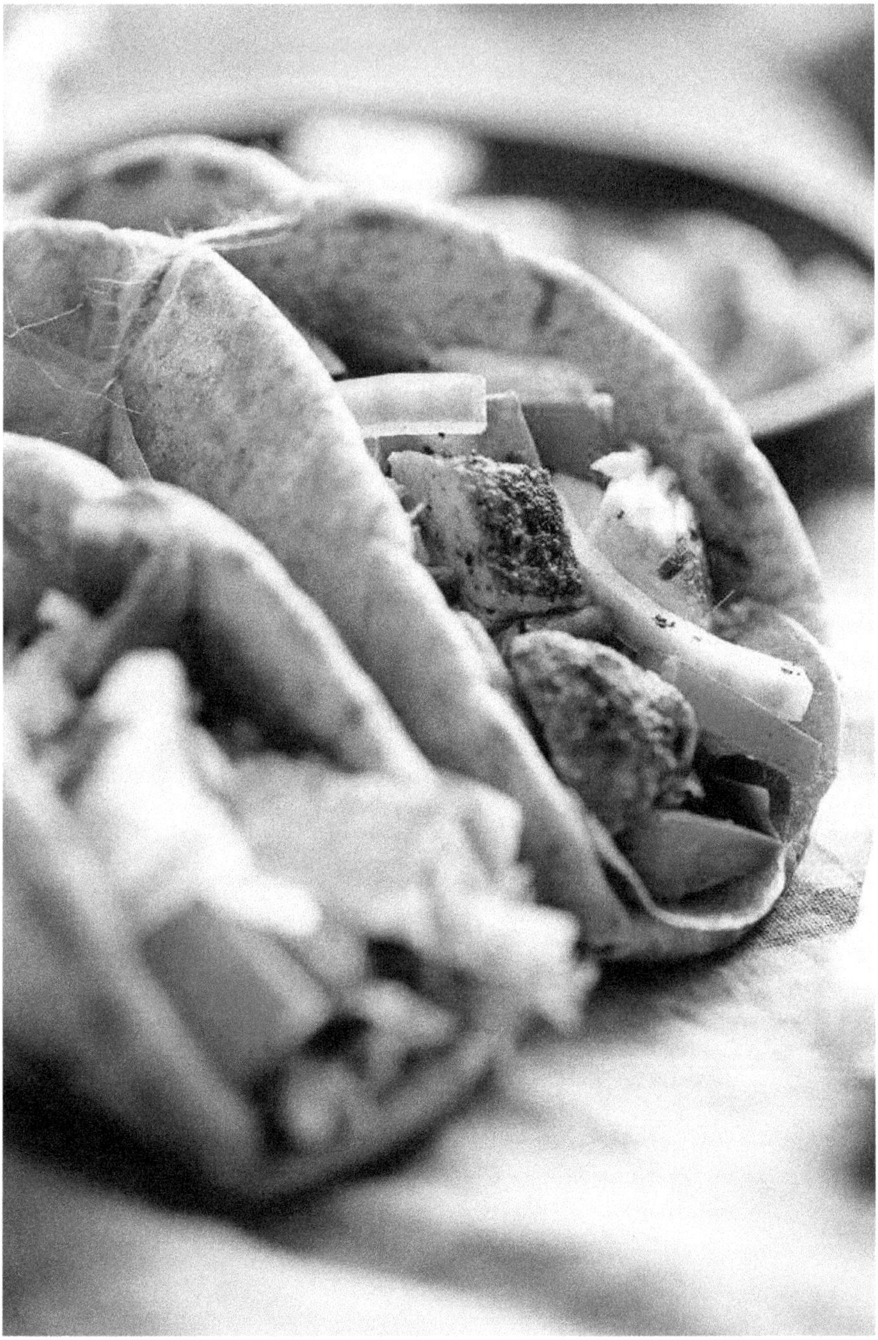

Chicken Shawarma

Ingredients:

- 2 lb. chicken breast, sliced into strips
- 1 teaspoon paprika
- 1 teaspoon ground cumin
- 1/4 teaspoon granulated garlic
- 1/2 teaspoon turmeric
- 1/4 teaspoon ground allspice

Directions

1. Season the chicken with spices and a little salt and pepper.
2. Pour 1 cup chicken broth to the skillet.
3. Seal the skillet.
4. Choose poultry setting.
5. Cook for 15 minutes.
6. Release the pressure naturally. Serve with flatbread.

Honey Balsamic Chicken

Ingredients:

- 1/4 cup honey
- 1/2 cup balsamic vinegar
- 1/4 cup soy sauce
- 2 cloves garlic minced
- 10 chicken drumsticks

Directions:

1. Mix the honey, vinegar, soy sauce and garlic in a bowl.
2. Soak the chicken in the sauce for 30 minutes.
3. Cover the skillet.
4. Set it to manual.
5. Cook at high pressure for 10 minutes.
6. Release the pressure quickly.
7. Choose the sauté button to thicken the sauce.

Garlic and Lemon Chicken Dish

Ingredients:

- 2-3 pounds chicken breast
- 1 teaspoon salt
- 1 onion, diced
- 1 tablespoon ghee
- 5 garlic cloves, minced
- ½ cup organic chicken broth
- 1 teaspoon dried parsley
- 1 large lemon, juiced
- 3-4 teaspoon arrowroot flour

Directions:

1. Set your skillet to Sauté mode. Add diced up the onion and cooking fat
2. Allow the onions to cook for 5 -10 minutes
3. Add the rest of the ingredients except arrowroot flour
4. Lock up the lid and set the skillet to poultry mode. Cook until the timer runs out
5. Allow the pressure to release naturally
6. Once done, remove ¼ cup of the sauce from the skillet and add arrowroot to make a slurry

7. Add the slurry to the skillet to make the gravy thick. Keep stirring well. Serve!

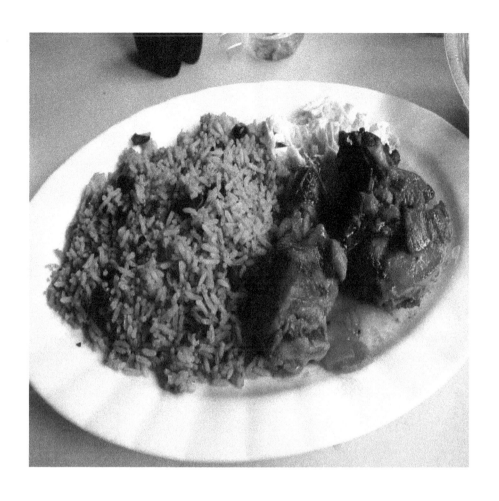

Belizean Chicken Stew

Ingredients:

- 4 whole chicken
- 1 tablespoon coconut oil
- 2 tablespoons achiote seasoning
- 2 tablespoons white vinegar
- 3 tablespoons Worcestershire sauce
- 1 cup yellow onion, sliced
- 3 garlic cloves, sliced
- 1 teaspoon ground cumin
- 1 teaspoon dried oregano
- ½ teaspoon black pepper
- 2 cups chicken stock

Directions:

1. Take a large-sized bowl and add achiote paste, vinegar, Worcestershire sauce, oregano, cumin and pepper. Mix well and add chicken pieces and rub the marinade all over them
2. Allow the chicken to sit overnight. Set your skillet to Sauté mode and add coconut oil
3. Once hot, cook chicken pieces to the skillet in batches. Remove the seared chicken and transfer them to a plate

4. Add onions, garlic to the skillet and Sauté for 2-3 minutes. Add chicken pieces back to the skillet
5. Pour chicken broth into the bowl with marinade and stir well. Add the mixture to the skillet.
6. Seal up the lid and cook for about 20 minutes at high pressure
7. Once done, release the pressure naturally. Season with a bit of salt and serve!

SOUP RECIPES

Veggie Barley Soup

Ingredients:

- 2 quarts of vegetable broth, 2 celery stalks, chopped
- 2 tall carrots, chopped
- 1 cup of barley
- Garbanzo beans, drained, 1 (15 ounce) can 1 chopped zucchini
- 1 (14.5 ounce) can of tomatoes containing juice
- 1 chopped onion
- 3 leaves from the bay
- 1 tsp. Parsley dried
- 1 tsp. White Sugar
- 1 tsp. Powdered garlic
- 1 tsp. Sauce from Worcestershire
- 1 tsp. Tweet Paprika
- 1 tsp. The Curry Powder
- 1/2 tsp. Yellow pepper on the ground
- For 1 tsp. The Salt of the Sea

Directions:

1. Add broth over medium heat to a large soup pot.

---

2. Stir together the celery, the carrots, the barley, the garbanzo beans, the zucchini, the peppers, the onion, the bay leaves, the parsley, the sugar, the garlic powder, the Worcestershire sauce, the paprika, the curry powder, the sea salt, the pepper.
3. Bring the mixture to a boil; cover and reduce the heat to medium-low heat.
4. Cook until the soup is thick or about 90 minutes.
5. Scrap the bay leaves and serve them sweet.

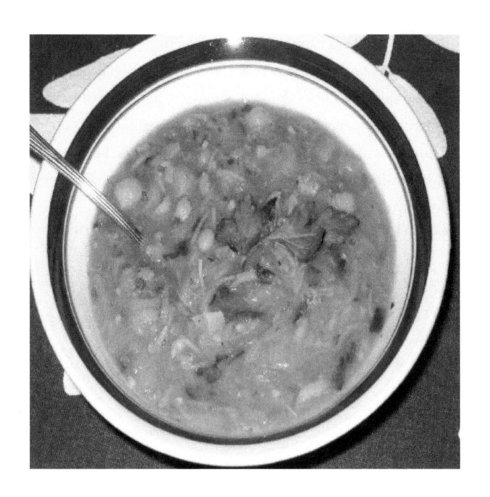

Chickpea Soup

Ingredients:

- 1 tbsp. Olive Oil Extra Virgin
- Garlic 4 cloves, minced
- 1 cup of onion diced
- 2 (15-oz.) cans of rinsed, drained chickpeas
- 1/4 cup of lemon juice, freshly squeezed
- 1/2 cup of parsley chopped
- 1 leaf of bay
- Tsp. 1 1/2. The Salt of the Sea
- Oil with Moroccan Spice

Direction:

1. In a medium saucepan set over medium heat, heat extra virgin olive oil; add garlic and onion and sauté, stirring, for 10 minutes or until browning begins. Four cups of water, chickpeas, parsley and bay leaf are added; stir and bring to a boil, filled with water.
2. Lower the heat and simmer for 15 minutes or so. Apply the sea salt and discard the bay leaves.
3. In batches, in a food processor, puree the soup until very thick and creamy.
4. Place the pureed soup back in the pan and add the lemon juice.

5. Drizzle with about half a teaspoon of Moroccan Spice Oil and sprinkle with parsley. Ladle the soup into bowls.

Red Lentil Bean Soup

Ingredients:

- 2 cups of dried, rinsed red lentil beans
- For 2 tbsp. For drizzling, extra virgin olive oil, plus more
- 2 big, diced onions
- 1 - 2 carrots that are finely chopped
- Chicken Stock 8 Cups
- 2 tomatoes, ripe, cubed
- For 1 tsp. Cumin from the ground
- Salt from the Sea
- Black Pepper
- 2 new cups of spinach

Directions:

1. For at least 2 hours, soak the lentils.
2. Boil the lentils in a pot placed over medium-high heat until nearly cooked. Heat extra virgin olive oil over medium heat in a soup pot; add the diced onions and carrots and sauté for approximately 4 minutes or until tender.
3. Add stock, tomatoes, cumin, sea salt and pepper and simmer until lentils are soft, or around 40 minutes.

4. Stir in spinach until wilted, and just before serving, drizzle with extra virgin olive oil.

Minestrone Soup

Ingredients:

- 1 small white onion
- 4 cloves garlic
- 1/2 cup carrots
- 1 medium zucchini
- 1 medium yellow squash
- 2 tablespoons minced fresh parsley
- 1/4 cup celery sliced
- 3 tablespoons olive oil
- 2 x 15 oz. cans cannellini beans
- 2 x 15 oz. can red kidney beans
- 1 x 14.5 oz. can fire-roasted diced tomatoes, drained
- 4 cups vegetable stock
- 2 cups of water
- 1 1/2 teaspoons oregano
- 1/2 teaspoon basil
- 1/4 teaspoon thyme
- 1 teaspoon salt
- 1/2 teaspoon pepper
- 3/4 cup small pasta shells
- 4 cups fresh baby spinach

- 1/4 cup Parmesan or Romano cheese

Directions:

1. Grab a stockpot and place over medium heat. Add the oil, then the onions, garlic, carrots, zucchini, squash, parsley, and celery. Cook for five minutes until the veggies are getting soft.

2. Pour in the stock, water, beans, tomatoes, herbs, and salt and pepper. Stir well. Decrease heat, cover, and simmer for 30 minutes.

3. Add the pasta and spinach, stir well, then cover and cook for a further 20 minutes until the pasta is cooked through. Stir through the cheese, then serve and enjoy.

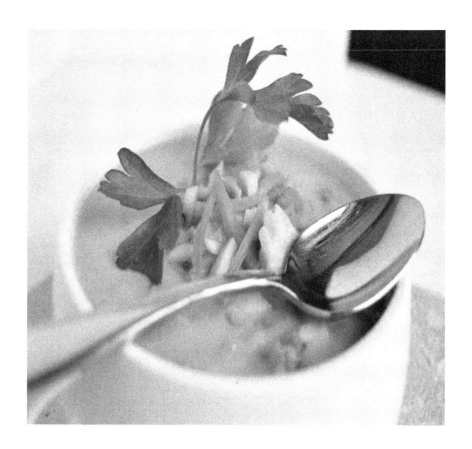

Chicken Wild Rice Soup

Ingredients:

- 2/3 cup wild rice, uncooked
- 1 tablespoon onion, chopped finely
- 1 tablespoon fresh parsley, chopped
- 1 cup carrots, chopped
- 8-ounces chicken breast, cooked
- 2 tablespoon butter
- 1/4 cup all-purpose white flour
- 5 cups low-sodium chicken broth
- 1 tablespoon slivered almonds

Directions:

1. Start by adding rice and 2 cups broth along with ½ cup water to a cooking pot. Cook the chicken until the rice is al dente and set it aside. Add butter to a saucepan and melt it.
2. Stir in onion and sauté until soft, then add the flour and the remaining broth.
3. Stir it and then cook for it 1 minute then add the chicken, cooked rice, and carrots. Cook for 5 minutes on simmer. Garnish with almonds. Serve fresh.

Classic Chicken Soup

Ingredients:

- 1 1/2 cups low-sodium vegetable broth
- 1 cup of water
- 1/4 teaspoon poultry seasoning
- 1/4 teaspoon black pepper
- 1 cup chicken strips
- 1/4 cup carrot
- 2-ounces egg noodles, uncooked

Directions:

1. Gather all the ingredients into a slow cooker and toss it cook soup on high heat for 25 minutes.
2. Serve warm.

Cucumber Soup

Ingredients:

- 2 medium cucumbers
- 1/3 cup sweet white onion
- 1 green onion
- 1/4 cup fresh mint
- 2 tablespoons fresh dill
- 2 tablespoons lemon juice
- 2/3 cup water
- 1/2 cup half and half cream
- 1/3 cup sour cream
- 1/2 teaspoon pepper
- Fresh dill sprigs for garnish

Directions:

1. Situate all of the ingredients into a food processor and toss. Puree the mixture and refrigerate for 2 hours. Garnish with dill sprigs. Enjoy fresh.

DESSERTS

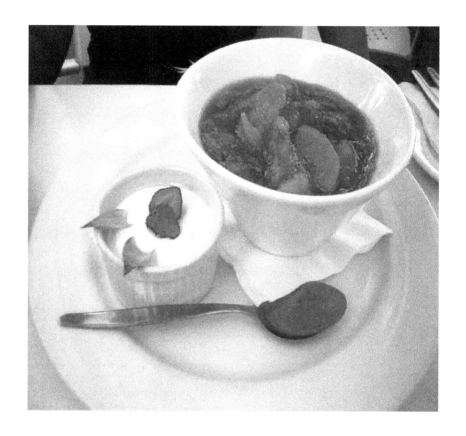

Vanilla Apple Compote

Ingredients:

- 3 cups apples, cored and cubed
- 1 tsp vanilla
- 3/4 cup coconut sugar
- 1 cup of water
- 2 tbsp fresh lime juice

Directions:

1. Add all ingredients into the inner pot of the instant pot and stir well.
2. Seal pot with lid and cook on high for 15 minutes.
3. Once done, allow to release pressure naturally for 10 minutes, then release remaining using quick release. Remove lid.
4. Stir and serve.

Apple Dates Mix

Ingredients:

- 4 apples, cored and cut into chunks
- 1 tsp vanilla
- 1 tsp cinnamon
- 1/2 cup dates, pitted
- 1 1/2 cups apple juice

Directions:

1. Add all ingredients into the inner pot of the instant pot and stir well.
2. Seal pot with lid and cook on high for 15 minutes.
3. Once done, allow to release pressure naturally for 10 minutes, then release remaining using quick release. Remove lid.
4. Stir and serve.

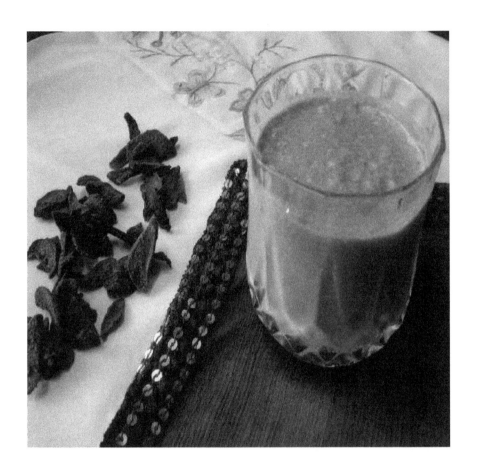

Choco Rice Pudding

Ingredients:

- 1 1/4 cup rice
- 1/4 cup dark chocolate, chopped
- 1 tsp vanilla
- 1/3 cup coconut butter
- 1 tsp liquid stevia
- 2 1/2 cups almond milk

Directions:

1. Add all ingredients into the inner pot of the instant pot and stir well.
2. Seal pot with lid and cook on high for 20 minutes.
3. Once done, allow to release pressure naturally. Remove lid.
4. Stir well and serve.

Grapes Stew

Ingredients:

- 1 cup grapes, halved
- 1 tsp vanilla
- 1 tbsp fresh lemon juice
- 1 tbsp honey
- 2 cups rhubarb, chopped
- 2 cups of water

Directions:

1. Add all ingredients into the inner pot of the instant pot and stir well.
2. Seal pot with lid and cook on high for 15 minutes.
3. Once done, allow to release pressure naturally for 10 minutes, then release remaining using quick release. Remove lid.
4. Stir and serve.

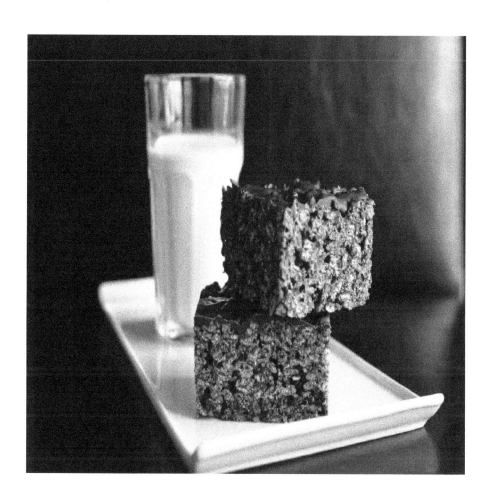

Chocolate Rice

Ingredients:

- 1 cup of rice
- 1 tbsp cocoa powder
- 2 tbsp maple syrup
- 2 cups almond milk

Directions:

1. Add all ingredients into the inner pot of the instant pot and stir well.
2. Seal pot with lid and cook on high for 20 minutes.
3. Once done, allow to release pressure naturally for 10 minutes, then release remaining using quick release. Remove lid.
4. Stir and serve.

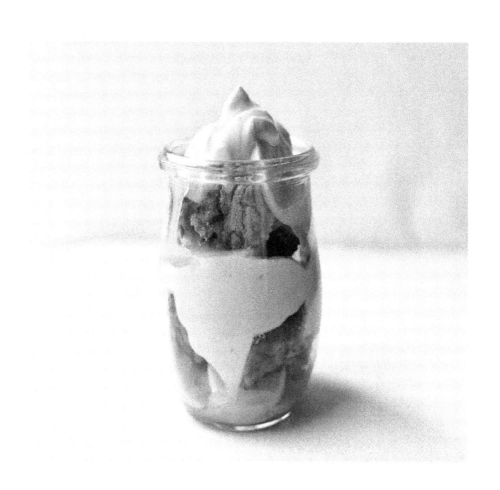

Vanilla Cream

Ingredients:

- 1 cup almond milk
- 1 cup coconut cream
- 2 cups coconut sugar
- 2 tablespoons cinnamon powder
- 1 teaspoon vanilla extract

Directions:

1. Heat a pan with the almond milk over medium heat, add the rest of the ingredients, whisk, and cook for 10 minutes more.
2. Divide the mix into bowls, cool down, and keep in the fridge for 2 hours before serving.

Blueberries Bowls

Ingredients:

- 1 teaspoon vanilla extract
- 2 cups blueberries
- 1 teaspoon coconut sugar
- 8 ounces Greek yogurt

Directions:

1.   Mix strawberries with the vanilla and the other ingredients, toss and serve cold.

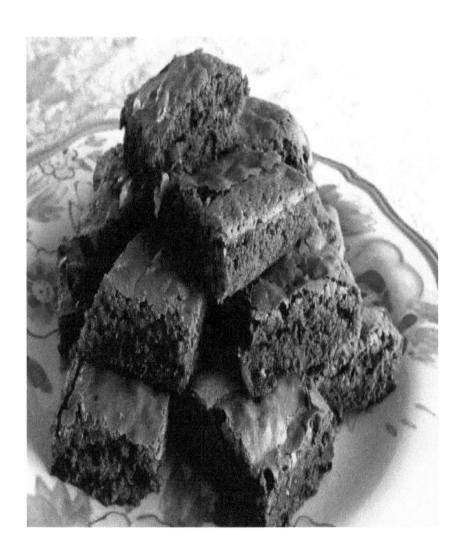

Brownies

Ingredients:

- 1 cup pecans, chopped
- 3 tablespoons coconut sugar
- 2 tablespoons cocoa powder
- 3 eggs, whisked
- ¼ cup avocado oil
- ½ teaspoon baking powder
- 2 teaspoons vanilla extract
- Cooking spray

Directions:

1. In your food processor, combine the pecans with the coconut sugar and the other ingredients except for the cooking spray and pulse well.
2. Grease a square pan with cooking spray, add the brownies mix, spread, introduce in the oven, bake at 350 degrees F for 25 minutes, leave aside to cool down, slice and serve.

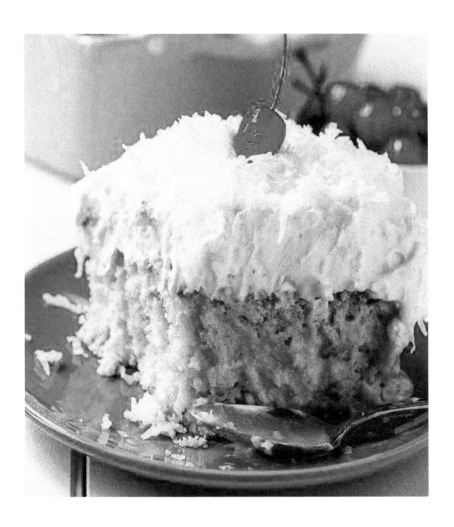

Strawberries Coconut Cake

Ingredients:

- 2 cups almond flour
- 1 cup strawberries, chopped
- ½ teaspoon baking soda
- ½ cup coconut sugar
- ¾ cup coconut milk
- ¼ cup avocado oil
- 2 eggs, whisked
- 1 teaspoon vanilla extract
- Cooking spray

Directions:

1. In a bowl, combine the flour with the strawberries and the other ingredients except the cooking spray and whisk well.
2. Grease a cake pan with cooking spray, pour the cake mix, spread, bake in the oven at 350 degrees F for 25 minutes, cool down, slice and serve.

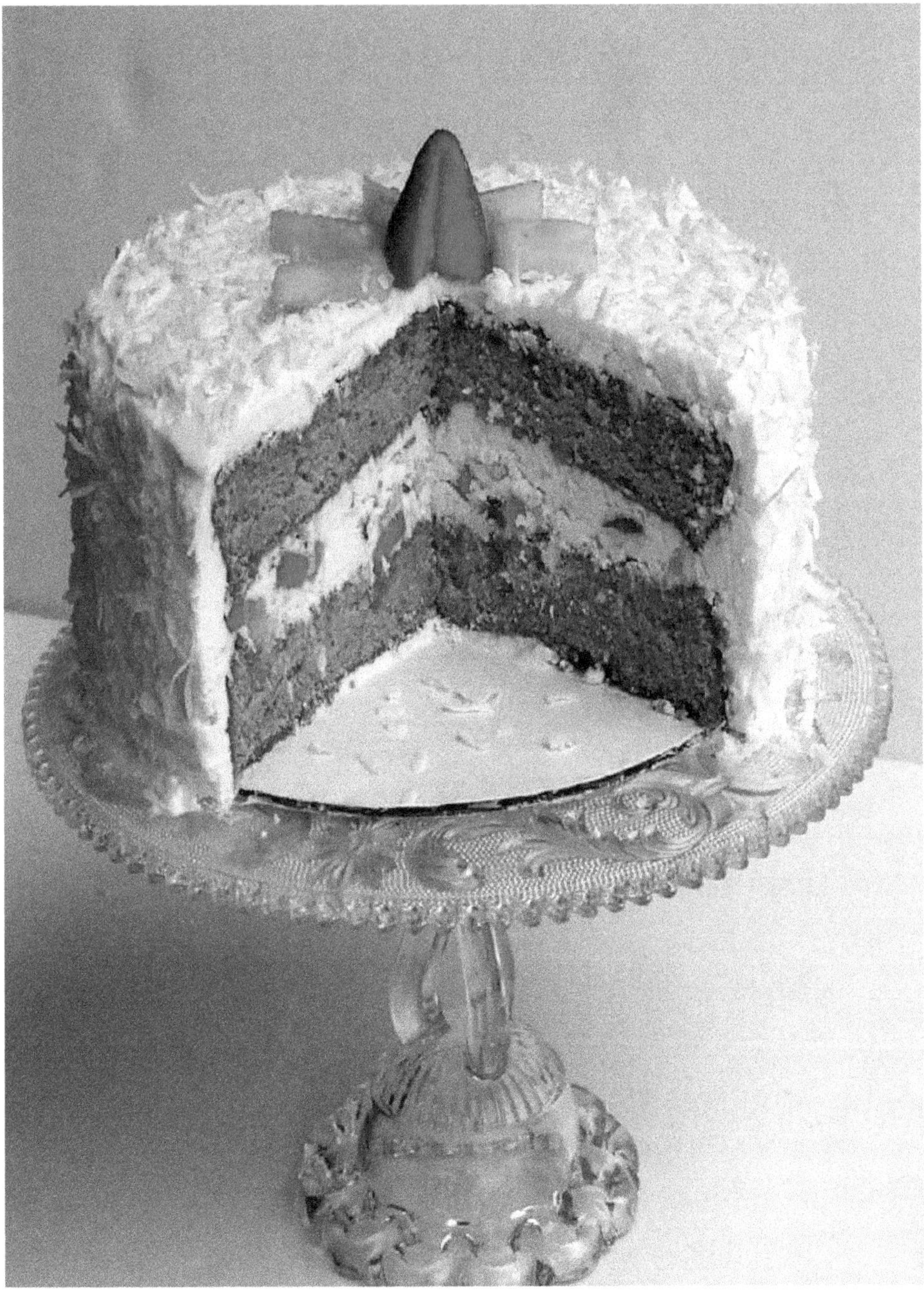

Cocoa Almond Pudding

Ingredients:

- 2 tablespoons coconut sugar
- 3 tablespoons coconut flour
- 2 tablespoons cocoa powder
- 2 cups almond milk
- 2 eggs, whisked
- ½ teaspoon vanilla extract

Directions:

1. Fill milk in a pan, add the cocoa and the other ingredients, whisk, simmer over medium heat for 10 minutes, pour into small cups, and serve cold.

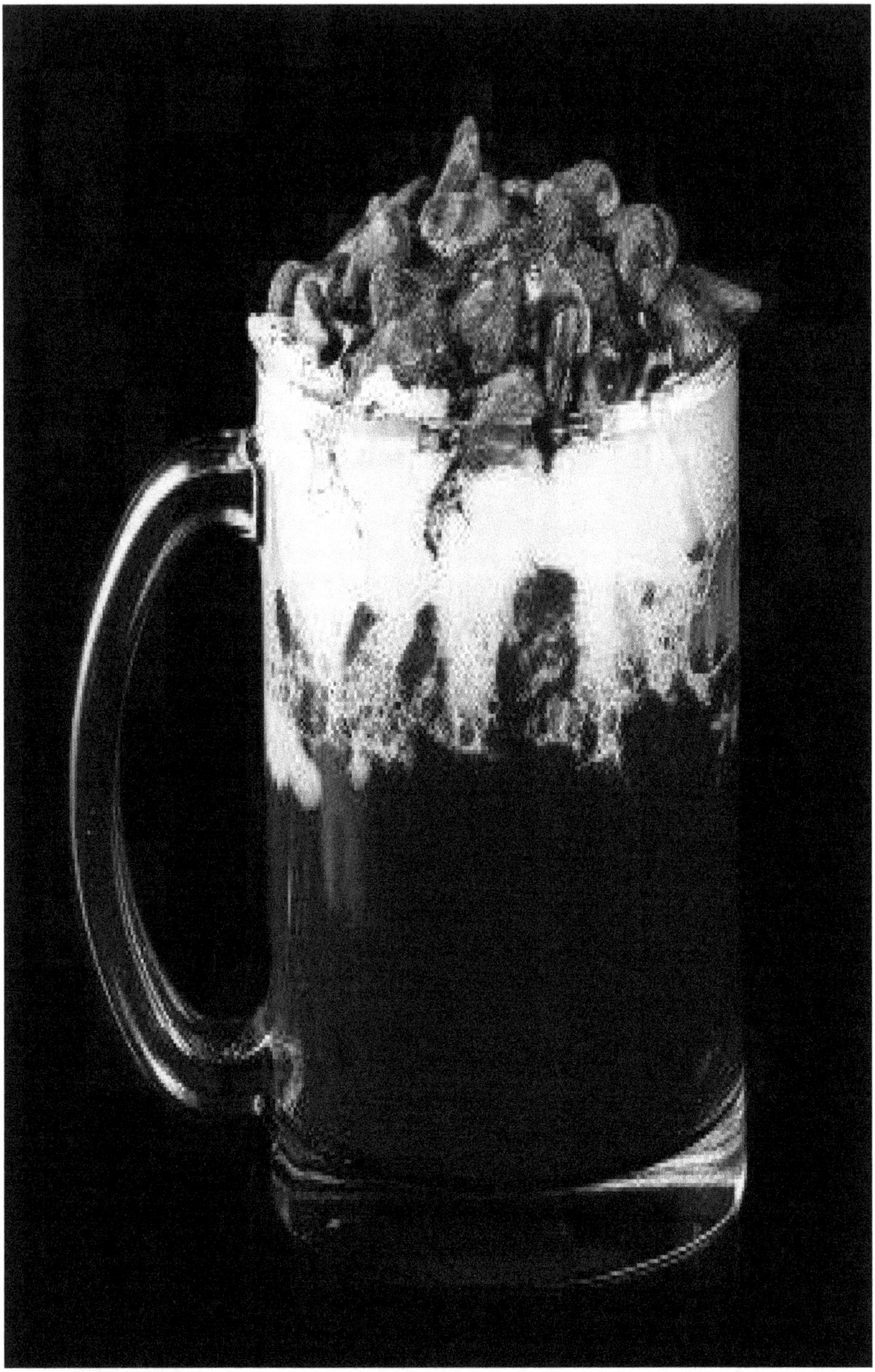

CPSIA information can be obtained
at www.ICGtesting.com
Printed in the USA
BVHW011710160321
602658BV00006B/311

9 781802 223750